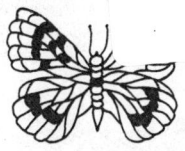

Cooking with Abstinence

Other Books by Lady Anne

FOR THE SEVERELY OBESE
GUIDE TO SPONSORING
HOW TO HELP SOMEONE YOU LOVE LOSE WEIGHT

LADY ANNE

Cooking with Abstinence

An Inspirational Cookbook for the Compulsive Overeater

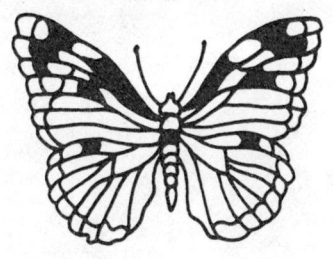

A DOLPHIN BOOK
DOUBLEDAY & COMPANY, INC.
GARDEN CITY, NEW YORK

1984

Library of Congress Cataloging in Publication Data
Anne, Lady.
Cooking with Abstinence.
"A Dolphin Book."
1. Cookery.   2. Reducing diets.   I. Title.
TX652.A56   1984   641.5'635

Library of Congress Catalog Card Number: 81–43898
ISBN 0-385-18140-X
Copyright © 1976, 1984 by LADY ANNE
Printed in the United States of America
All rights reserved

First Edition

Contents

GUIDE TO WEIGHTS AND MEASURES

1	Good Morning	3
2	Luncheon	14
3	Dinner	29
4	Entertaining	49
5	Salads and Vegetables	54
6	Specialties: Desserts, "Free" Dressing, Relishes, Treats	76
7	Just for Today	83
8	The Butterfly Story	85

Dedication

To my Sponsors and friends in Program who gave me love when I could not love myself, who took an ugly creature and found something of worth and taught me to value myself and to love others. To all compulsive overeaters who understood.

All that I have, all that I am, all that I ever hope to be, I owe to God through my Program.

Partnership

Together . . . . . . we can

God

*My
Higher
Power, my
Program and
my action, have
taken off in these
twelve months 175 lbs. +
with my compulsion arrested,
through abstinence, I am able to
work on the emotional and spiritual.*

My Action   Program

Author's Note

Today, after being in Program a year and being totally abstinent on gray sheet, I can honestly say that I have enjoyed my meals without guilt, have never felt bored or deprived. Why? It's simple . . . I have accepted that I am a compulsive overeater, always was, always will be. There are some things in life I will not be able to have, but the things I can have I have enjoyed and will continue to do so. It is my right as a human being to give myself enjoyment.

My disease presents enough inconveniences without adding a self-imposed punishment. I am not a criminal sentencing myself to a life of imprisonment, I am not bearing the guilt of an unforgivable sin, therefore, penance is inappropriate. I am not "a bad person getting good, I am a sick person getting well."

To say that food is not important to me would be dishonest and my program teaches my honesty. No, I do not look forward to food with great anticipation. No, food is not the most important thing in my life. No, I don't think food should be mentioned at the meetings.

AUTHOR'S NOTE

Abstinence is the most important thing in my life without exception. I practice "301." Three meals a day with nothing in between, one day at a time. I plan on practicing "301" for the rest of my life, one day at a time. I can't afford to get bored with food. That would be a setup to fail and I have no desire to feel deprived or to fail. I'm much too happy, comfortable, or serene, if you will.

Many of my program friends have eaten at my house and have been surprised at the fact that they have dined and enjoyed themselves, and were amazed at how "normal" they felt.

I have shared recipes with them, but mostly, I have shared attitude.

Since so many of my friends have asked me for recipes I thought I might put them together in this book, as a service, as a labor of love.

My first recipe is for a "Magic Formula." It goes like this:

1 cup of awareness

2 cups of attitude

3 cups of action

Mix well and add (according to taste) meetings, telephone calls, literature, writing, service, sponsors, and cover with anonymity for a lifetime, one day at a time, and you will come up with the most beautiful *abstinence*.

Abstinence is the most delicious thing you have ever "tasted." And, it feels comfortable, lasts longer, and looks terrific. And if that isn't enough, abstinence gives you acceptance of yourself, of others and your acceptance gives *Serenity*.

So, I'll Repeat:

Awareness + *Attitude* + *Action* =

Abstinence = *Acceptance* = *Serenity*

I pray that you find the material on the following pages helpful as the intent of this work is to give service and responsible love to those of you who have given to me, in the past, now, and in the next "24."

WARNING: I am not an authority, nor am I writing this book as an authority. Check with your sponsor and always remember . . . When in DOUBT, *leave it OUT.* Approach with vigilance.

If any of these recipes become a potential binge food and the warning signals starts to flash . . . Let Go.

Happy Abstinence.
Love,
Lady Anne

GUIDE TO WEIGHTS AND MEASURES

*God grant me
the Serenity to Accept
the things I cannot change,
Courage to change the things I can,
and Wisdom to know the difference.*

TABLE I:
A GUIDE TO WEIGHTS AND MEASURES

1 teaspoon = 60 drops
3 teaspoons = 1 tablespoon
2 tablespoons = 1 fluid ounce
4 tablespoons = 1/4 cup
5 1/3 tablespoons = 1/3 cup
8 tablespoons = 1/2 cup
16 tablespoons = 1 cup
1 pound = 16 ounces
1 cup = 1/2 pint
2 cups = 1 pint
4 cups = 1 quart
4 quarts = 1 gallon

STANDARD ABBREVIATIONS

t. — teaspoon
T. — tablespoon
c. — cup
pt. — pint
d. — drop

qt. — quart
d.b. — double boiler
oz. — ounce
lb. — pound

1
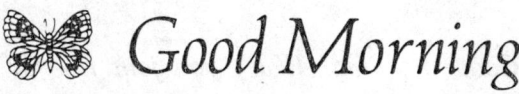 Good Morning

Through Discipline We Find Freedom

"I strongly suggest not using eye judgment but weighing and measuring food." This is a practice of good cooks everywhere, for the compulsive overeater, a necessary discipline.

"Compulsive overeaters are not bad people trying to get good . . . we are sick people trying to get well."

Good morning! Won't you join me for a delicious, abstinent breakfast?

BREAKFAST SUGGESTIONS

- **EGG PIZZA**

(1 PROTEIN)
1 egg
½ t. onion flakes
Salt and pepper
½ oz. mozzarella cheese
Dash of oregano

TO PREPARE: Beat egg, add onion flakes, salt and pepper. Pour into a small pan (preheated and coated with non-stick spray). Cook for approximately 1 minute, turn, lay on strips of cheese, sprinkle with oregano, cover pan. Cook 2 minutes on lowered flame.
Try this with different cheese for variety.

- **PANCAKE**

(1 PROTEIN)
1 egg
2 oz. farmer cheese
Sweetener (to taste, suggest ½ packet)
Dash of salt

(1 FRUIT PORTION)
Serve with Blueberry Sauce: ½ c. blueberries
1 packet sweetener
2 T. cold water

Mix ingredients, cook in small pot, bring to boil. Serve over pancake.

TO PREPARE: Combine ingredients in blender and mix until you have smooth batter. Preheat flat pan and coat with nonstick spray. Pour batter, cook until light brown, turn, and finish cooking on other side. Should resemble real pancake.

Just for today, I'll be as happy as I can.

• SCRAMBLED EGG SUPREME

(1 PROTEIN)
1 egg
1 1/2 oz. cottage cheese
2 oz. milk

TO PREPARE: Combine and beat ingredients, add salt and pepper (to taste), pour into preheated non-stick pan, scramble, and cook 3 minutes.

Today I shall practice HALT. I will not allow myself to get too Hungry, too Angry, too Lonely, or too Tired.

• PIGLETS 'N' EGG

(1 PROTEIN)
1 hot dog
1 egg
Dash of onion flakes
Dash garlic powder
Salt and pepper

TO PREPARE: Cut hot dog into ¼-in. rings, sauté in two drops oil. Add egg, seasoning, and scramble. Cook hot dog until brown on both sides, then cook another minute after adding egg.

- **COMPLETE BLENDER BREAKFAST**

(1 PROTEIN + 1 FRUIT PORTION)
8 oz. milk
1 egg
2 d. vanilla
Dash nutmeg
1 c. strawberries
1 packet sweetener

TO PREPARE: Combine ingredients in blender, about 1 minute. Yield: 2 glasses, very filling.

Lord, help me find gray or moderation in my life. Not just the extremes.

EGG ROLLS

(1 PROTEIN)
1 egg
1 strip bacon, cooked and crumbled
½ oz. grated cheese
Salt and pepper (to taste)

TO PREPARE: Beat egg and pour into pan with bacon drippings. Make sure egg covers bottom of entire pan so it will be thin. Add bacon, cheese, and season. Lower flame and cook until cheese starts to melt. Roll up and serve hot.

Abstinence from Compulsive Overeating Is the Most Important Thing in My Life Without Exception. Abstinence from Negative Thinking Is a Close Second. Today, Lord, let me see the "Glass Half Full, not Half Empty."

- **BLINTZ ENGLISH STYLE**

(1 PROTEIN)
Margarine
1 egg (beat well)
¼ c. cottage cheese (or farmer or ricotta)
1 t. lemon juice
Sweetener to taste

TO PREPARE: Coat small frying pan with margarine, spread egg thinly, and cook until firm, 2 minutes. Then place on dish, add cheese, roll up. Top with lemon juice and sprinkle with sweetener. Very nice. *Try this with your fruit portion of berries sometime for complete breakfast.

SPECIAL BREAKFAST SUGGESTIONS

- **PINEAPPLE CHEESE DELIGHT**

(1 PROTEIN + 1 FRUIT PORTION)
½ c. ricotta cheese
1 c. pineapple
Dash of cinnamon
Sweetener (optional)

TO PREPARE: Just mix gently and enjoy. Fast, delicious, and an excellent meal to take to anywhere if you're planning to eat breakfast out. Very filling and refreshing.

Use pineapple chunks packed in water if fresh pineapple is not available. Also, try this same combination using ½ c. strawberries and ½ c. pineapple for variety.

This Day Is Mine. What I do with it is up to me and no one else. The choice is mine, I can use it for good or squander it away. Lord, help me not regret its passing as it will never come again.

- **CHICKEN LIVERS WITH BACON**

(1 PROTEIN)
2 oz. cooked chicken livers*
2 strips cooked bacon (crumbled)
Onion flakes
Sage
Thyme
Salt and pepper

*Chicken livers may be boiled ahead of time and kept in container in refrigerator for convenient use.

TO PREPARE: Place livers in bacon drippings in a heated pan with onion flakes, sprinkle with seasoning, add bacon, and turn several times. Lower flame, cover, and cook for 3 minutes. Serve hot.

A citrus fruit such as 1 orange, or ½ grapefruit, or 2 tangerines is a nice combination with this menu. Top off with cinnamon coffee (see below).

CINNAMON COFFEE: Just prepare coffee as usual. For an unusual change, add a cinnamon stick and sweetener to taste. Serve black and hot.

Together . . . We Can. "One Day, One Pound at a Time."

• LADY ANNE'S "TREAT YOURSELF LIKE COMPANY" BREAKFAST

(1 PROTEIN + 1 FRUIT PORTION)
2 oz. cooked bacon
½ c. pineapple chunks (packed in own juice)
Dash cinnamon
½ apple, peeled and diced
Dash ginger
1 t. lemon juice
1 slice ham, 2 oz.

TO PREPARE: In hot bacon fat, add ½ c. pineapple with cinnamon, brown for minute, turning so that it does not stick. Add diced apple, sprinkle with ginger, add lemon juice, and cook until apple is starting to get tender. Add ham. Cook on each side about one minute. Place bacon slices on top; cover for about ½ minute. Serve hot.

Serve a Cup of HOT BLACK 'N' ORANGE

Prepare pot of coffee and add 2 drops of orange extract to the pot after it has perked and let stand for a minute before serving. It is a delightful treat. Add sweetener according to taste.

Thank you for sharing breakfast with me. It's so much more fun together . . . Keep Coming Back.

It Is Chance
That Makes Brothers
But Hearts
That Make Friends.
        LORD LESTER

2

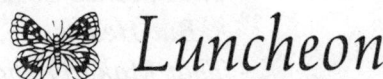 *Luncheon*

Paradox: *"We Give that we may live"*
Paradox: *"Only the losers win"*
Paradox: *"We surrender to be free"*
Paradox: *"We die in order to live"*

You're invited to examine and try the recipes on the next pages. Remember . . . ATTITUDE; how you approach your meals could mean the difference between a happy abstinence or struggle and defeat. How *we serve* as well as What *we serve* is important. It is my opinion that compulsive people are very creative people. So . . . BE CREATIVE . . . ENJOY.

- **TUNA BOAT**

½ c. tuna
1 cucumber
⅛ c. diced carrots (raw)
⅛ c. diced raw onion
½ c. diced pickle artificially presweetened
4 radishes
1 tomato
Lemon juice

TO PREPARE: Hold cucumber lengthwise and slice about ½ inch from side. Scoop out center and place on dish so cuke resembles a canoe. Mix tuna with carrots, onion, pickle, and lemon juice in bowl, then fill the cucumber "boat." Place the slice of cucumber you first cut off on two toothpicks and put a roof on your boat. Garnish with radishes, and tomato wedges which can be eaten with cucumber boat as a finger salad. This is a complete luncheon. It is very attractive and very good-tasting. Try it with program people and watch the expression on their faces.

Paradox: When I accept myself, just as I am, then I can change.

Rogers

LUNCHEON

- **DEVILED EGG AND TUNA DELIGHTS**

(1 PROTEIN = 1 FINGER SALAD)
1 hard-boiled egg
2 oz. tuna
½ t. mustard
¼ t. onion flakes
Garlic powder
Salt and pepper to taste
Lettuce leaves
Paprika and parsley flakes
Tomato slices
(plus ½ c. beets = 1 veg.)

TO PREPARE: Slice egg in half lengthwise; scoop out yolk. Mix yolk, tuna, mustard, onion flakes, dash of garlic powder, salt and pepper in bowl. Fill center of egg whites. Place on lettuce leaves. Sprinkle with paprika and parsley flakes. Serve with tomato slices and ½ c. beets.

HOW?

So many beginners ask me how I work my program. My answer to them sounds like double-talk. I say, "Yes, that is how I work my program, by practicing HOW."
Honesty + Openmindedness + Willingness

OMELETS . . . OMELETS . . . OMELETS . . .

- **WESTERN**

(1 PROTEIN + ½ VEG.)
1 egg
2 oz. cubed ham
⅛ c. diced onion
¼ c. diced raw green pepper

TO PREPARE: Beat egg, add other ingredients, pour into small, lightly greased pan. Turn after egg gets firm on bottom side. Cook with cover so egg can fluff. Serve hot.

- **ZIPPY CHEESE**

(1 PROTEIN)
1 egg
2 d. mustard
Salt and pepper to taste
Dash of onion flakes
Margarine
Cheese (1 oz. of American, Swiss, or other hard cheese)

TO PREPARE: Combine ingredients except for cheese, and beat gently. Pour into heated frying pan coated lightly with margarine. When egg is just firming, lay cheese strips on half of egg and with spatula, fold the other half of egg over side covered with cheese. Cook about 2 minutes. Serve hot.

- **SPANISH OMELET**

(1 PROTEIN + ½ VEG.)
Margarine
2 eggs, well beaten
2 T. canned crushed tomato
2 T. diced green pepper
⅛ c. raw minced onion
Dash of Tabasco
Salt and pepper to taste

TO PREPARE: Coat small pan with margarine. Combine ingredients and pour into pan. Cook on one side until firm, gently turn, and cover. Finish cooking. Do not change the amount of the vegetable ingredients to equal your entire portion of vegetable. You will overwhelm the egg and not enjoy this delicious dish.

EASY DOES IT AND KEEP IT SIMPLE
This is not an easy Program and no one ever told me it would be easy, but they told me it was a simple one as long as I keep it that way for myself. One way I'm learning to "Keep It Simple" is to remember, often, to Utilize and not Analyze . . .

OTHER DELICIOUS OMELET SUGGESTIONS

ASPARAGUS   MUSHROOM   SPINACH
ZUCCHINI   PEPPERS   BROCCOLI

These omelets are excellent if you don't try to combine your entire vegetable portion in with the egg. Learn to subdivide, and the effort will be worth it.

- **PEPPERONI AND EGG**
  SAUSAGE AND EGG

(1 PROTEIN)
1 egg + 2 oz. meat, cooked as you would any omelet. It's a nice change. Just remember to dice the meat into very small pieces. Happy Omelets . . .

QUICKIE LUNCHES

Suggestions: For quickie lunches it is always a good idea to have cooked vegetables on hand in the refrigerator. I try to have as standards: string beans, zucchini, eggplant, cauliflower, broccoli, mushrooms, and peppers.

Awareness

Melted cheese over these vegetables is delicious and fast. For instance, 2 oz. cheese melted over a vegetable takes two minutes in the oven.

TRY: CAULIFLOWER & CHEDDAR & OR BROCCOLI & SWISS
½ C. STRING BEANS & ½ C. TOMATO & AMERICAN
EGGPLANT & RICOTTA OR MOZZARELLA

TO PREPARE: Cut eggplant into very thin slices. Place on baking sheet with tomato sauce seasoned with salt and pepper. Turn after 3 minutes, place back in oven, and cook 2 minutes. Three slices eggplant + ¼ c. tomato sauce is a 1-cup veg. Put away to use for many different meals. Use as base for "lasagne" or "pizza" or a one-dish casserole.

Attitude

LUNCHEON 21

• EGGPLANT ITALIAN

(1 PROTEIN + 1 VEG.)
3 slices prepared eggplant (as above)
2 oz. ricotta cheese
Italian seasoning
1 oz. mozzarella cheese
Tomato sauce

TO PREPARE: Use an individual baking dish and lay the eggplant on lightly greased surface; add ricotta, season to taste, cook 2 minutes. Add mozzarella and sauce. Cook 1 more minute in oven.

Action

• EGGPLANT LASAGNE—OVEN DISH

(1 PROTEIN + 1 VEG.)
Olive oil
1/4 c. tomato sauce
Sliced eggplant, precooked (p. 20)
1 1/2 oz. precooked beef or sausage
1 1/2 oz. ricotta cheese
1/2 oz. mozzarella cheese
Basil, oregano, salt, pepper, 1/2 packet sweetener

TO PREPARE: In individual pan, place 2 d. olive oil, 1 t. tomato sauce, lay 1 slice of eggplant flat. Add meat. Cover with second slice of eggplant, 1 t. tomato sauce. Add ricotta, and cover with third slice of eggplant. Add the remainder of tomato sauce. Season to taste, cook 4 minutes. Then place mozzarella to top off, and cook another minute. Delicious and filling.

- **PIZZA CON EGGPLANT**

(1 PROTEIN + 1 VEG.)
2 oz. pepperoni
1 oz. mozzarella cheese
Sliced eggplant, precooked (p. 20)
¼ c. tomato sauce
Oregano
Salt and pepper
Garlic powder

TO PREPARE: Weigh and divide your pepperoni and cheese into 3 even amounts as you will be spreading this on top of three slices of eggplant. Add tomato sauce and season generously. Bake in oven for 4 minutes at 350°. Cook on baking sheet lightly greased.

I'm not all that I should be, I'm not all that I could be, I'm not all that I want to be, but for the Grace of God, I'm not what I once was. (And I'm getting better everyday.)

• FISH 'N' CHIPS

(1 PROTEIN + ½ VEG.)
½ lb. Turbot
Margarine
2 d. lemon
Paprika
Onion flakes
Oregano
½ c. cucumber chips
¼ c. white vinegar
1 packet sweetener
Mint

TO PREPARE: Place turbot in flat pan with 1 t. margarine; add lemon juice and seasonings. Cover generously with paprika. Bake in oven at 350° for 15 minutes. Cucumber chips should be soaking in vinegar, sweetener and mint. When fish is done, weigh out 4 oz. for yourself and top with cucumber.

*Make enough for your family. It is very economical, and even the non-fish eaters like it.

Helen Keller said, "Life is a Banquet and most of us are Starving to Death." Today we can get fuller and higher than when we were overeating. Get full on love and the real things God provides for our needs.

- **SHRIMP CHOW MEIN**

(1 PROTEIN + 1 VEG. + 1 FINGER SALAD)
½ c. chopped raw onion
½ c. chopped raw celery
1 t. margarine
Salt and pepper
½ c. sliced mushrooms
4 oz. precooked shrimp

TO PREPARE: Cook onion in water and measure out ¼ cup. Sauté celery in 1 t. margarine, add salt, pepper, measure out ¼ cup. Cook separately mushrooms and add together all ingredients in fry pan and cook for a couple of minutes.

Take 1 cup of stripped crisp lettuce leaves, pour shrimp and vegetables over it, and enjoy.

• FANCY HOT DOG

(1 PROTEIN + 1 VEG.)
1 broiled hot dog
1 slice cooked bacon
½ oz. Swiss cheese
¼ c. chopped cooked onion
¼ c. tomato sauce
¼ c. chopped cooked peppers

TO PREPARE: Wrap bacon around hot dog, cover with cheese, and place in oven until cheese begins to melt, add rest of ingredients for 1 minute. Serve hot.

• HAMBURGER PIZZA

(1 PROTEIN + 1 VEG.)
5 oz. uncooked ground beef (weight after cooking 4 oz.)
½ c. tomato sauce
¼ c. raw onion
1 clove minced garlic
⅛ t. oregano
⅛ t. basil
Salt and pepper to taste
½ oz. mozzarella cheese strips

TO PREPARE: Add to hamburger meat ½ of the tomato sauce. Add ingredients except cheese. Shape into a patty and cook on grill or oven, turn, and add cheese ½ minute before burger is done. Add remainder of sauce and serve hot.

LUNCHEON

• MINUTE STEAK SURPRISE

(1 PROTEIN + 1 VEG.)
1 pat margarine
5 oz. raw steak (cooks down to 4 oz.)
½ t. onion flakes
¼ c. chopped peppers
¼ c. sliced mushrooms
¼ c. diced pickle

TO PREPARE: Cook all together in fry pan in 1 pat margarine for 10 minutes. Add seasoning to taste.

Be as good to yourself as you would be to your friend . . . You count too!

• CHICKEN LIVER SAUTÉ

(1 PROTEIN + 1 VEG. + 1 FINGER SALAD)
1 pat margarine
4 oz. fresh chicken livers
½ c. chopped raw onion (yield ¼ c. cooked)
Sage, thyme, oregano, garlic powder, salt and pepper

TO PREPARE: Melt margarine in frying pan and add chicken livers and seasonings, on high flame stirring so they won't stick. Brown and turn, lower flame, cook 15 minutes. Add onion about 2 minutes before removing from heat so it will be tender, not soggy.

Serve over bed of lettuce with a few drops of vinegar. The juice of the livers mixed with vinegar seems to dress the lettuce. Try this with ½ c. of sliced mushrooms. This is a complete meal.

- **STUFFED PEPPER**

(1 PROTEIN + 1 VEG.)
5 oz. raw ground beef (yield 4 oz. cooked)
¼ c. tomato sauce
¼ c. diced mushrooms
1 t. onion flakes
2 green pepper halves, seeds removed
Salt and pepper
Oregano
½ package sweetener
Basil

TO PREPARE: Mix beef with other ingredients and fill pepper. Place in 350° oven for 30 minutes in roasting pan with 1 inch of water.

- **STUFFED CABBAGE**

Parboil cabbage. Follow same recipe as above, using cabbage instead of pepper. Just add 1 t. vinegar.

"The smaller I get, the more of me there is to love."

3
Dinner

*Yesterday is history
Tomorrow a mystery,
All we have is today . . .
Let's make it beautiful.*

SEAFOOD SUPPERS

- **SWEET AND SOUR COLD FISH**

(4 OZ. = 1 PROTEIN)
4 pieces of pike or whitefish or salmon (or comb.)
3/4 c. water
1/4 c. white vinegar
1 c. onion flakes

1 T. sweetener
Salt and pepper
12 bay leaves
12 cloves

TO PREPARE: Boil in pot ¾ c. water plus vinegar, onion flakes, and sweetener. After water has boiled for 2 minutes, add salt and pepper to taste. Place fish in pan and pour water mixture over it. Mixture should just cover fish. Place cloves and bay leaves in cheesecloth, tie together so nothing comes out. Place in corner of pot and finish cooking fish for another 15 minutes. Take fish out, drain, and refrigerate. This fish will keep in refrigerator for two weeks. So convenient and so good. Just measure out your portion and enjoy.

- **GEFILTE FISH**

(3 ¾ OZ. = 1 PROTEIN)
2 lbs. whitefish
2 eggs
¼ c. water
Horseradish
Salt and pepper to taste
½ c. onion flakes
2 onions
2 carrots

TO PREPARE: Grind fish with onion flakes (some fish markets will do it for you). Chop fish in wooden bowl, adding 1 egg at a time (keep chopping) and then water and seasoning until mixture is the consistency of oatmeal. Shape mixture into flat loaves. Bring ⅓ pot of water to boil, adding the onions, carrots, and fish bones (for flavor only!). Boil for 5 minutes, remove fish bones, and place loaves in pot. Cover. Cook slowly for 2 hours, then drain and chill.

SUGGESTION: Keep hands moist while making fish loaves. Measure out 3 3/4 oz. for protein portion. Remember, we added egg. It's work, but worth it.

Abstinence isn't vanity, Abstinence is sanity.

- **STUFFED CLAMS**

(YIELD 2 PORTIONS)
1 dozen raw clams (small) = 4 oz.
1 pat margarine
1 T. diced onions
2 T. diced mushrooms
Clove garlic, crushed
2 T. diced celery
1 egg (beaten)
2 T. diced green pepper
1 T. wheat germ
Salt, pepper, oregano, horseradish (to taste)

TO PREPARE: Open clams and save both shells (24 shells). Dice clams, mix with all ingredients, and spoon into 24 clam shells. Place on cookie sheet in oven broiler for 10 minutes. Serve hot. Twelve stuffed clams on 1/2 shell = 1 portion and 1/2 veg. Reheat other 12 clams for a fast lunch next day.

- **STUFFED SOLE**

(1 PORTION + 3/4 VEG.)
Egg (beaten)
Dash of soy sauce, salt, pepper, oregano (to taste)
1 oz. crab meat
2 T. diced dill pickle
2 T. crushed tomato
1 T. wheat germ
1/2 c. vinegar
1 pat margarine, melted
1 packet sweetener
1 sprig mint, crushed

TO PREPARE: Mix 1/2 of beaten egg with seasoning, crab meat, pickle, tomato, and wheat germ. Spoon onto fillet and roll. Tie with string and place in oven at 350°. Bake about 15 minutes. While fish is cooking, pour 1/2 c. vinegar into cup, add margarine, sweetener, and mint. This makes a delicious sauce to pour over fish. You have 1/4 of a 1-cup vegetable coming. Try 2 T. of diced beets on your salad.

Recovery Is Learning to Cope with Living.

- **BAKED BLUE FISH**

(4 OZ. = 1 PROTEIN + ½ VEG.)
1 small fish, cleaned and boned
Seasoning to taste: oregano, salt and pepper, parsley flakes, thyme
¼ c. onion rings
¼ c. crushed tomato
¼ c. diced dill pickle
2 T. onion flakes
¼ t. paprika
1 pat margarine

TO PREPARE: Place fish on foil-covered baking pan and season. Add onion rings, tomato, pickle and onion flakes. Sprinkle paprika on last and add pat of margarine on top. Cook 20 minutes in oven at 375°. Serve hot.
There will be enough for a dinner companion too.

Become the one you Dream you can be.

• BOILED WHITIES WITH DILL

(4 oz. = 1 protein)
1 lb. whitefish
1 c. water
1 clove garlic
1 t. fresh dill
½ lemon
1 t. oil
Parsley flakes
Salt and pepper

TO PREPARE: Place fish in water, add other ingredients, including the unsqueezed ½ lemon, and boil for about 20 minutes. Delicious hot or served the next day cold with a little vinegar. Weigh out your portion and share with your family. They will like it, too.

SUGGESTION: This dish is complemented when served with ½ cup beets or carrots.

• STUFFED TOMATO WITH SHRIMP

(1 PROTEIN + ½ VEG.)
1 large ripe tomato
¼ t. basil
¼ t. onion flakes
½ packet sweetener
Salt and pepper to taste
4 oz. parboiled shrimp
1 pat margarine

¼ t. oregano
¼ t. mint leaves

TO PREPARE: Cut top off tomato and scoop out some of center. (Leave enough of a "wall"). Mix scooped portion of tomato with diced shrimp and all ingredients. Place in baking pan with 1 inch of water. Put in oven at 350° for 30 minutes. Serve hot.

Proverb:
What you get by dishonesty will do you no good,
but honesty can save your Life . . .
SOLOMON

- **STEAMERS**

(APPROX. 16 TO 4 OZ.)
Steamers
1 c. water
2 crushed garlic cloves
1 T. olive oil
Salt and pepper

TO PREPARE: Wash steamers (make sure shells are closed) and place in large pot with other ingredients. Cover and cook for 45 minutes. Steamers will make their own broth for dipping. Delicious. Make plenty for family.

DINNER

- **MUSSELS WITH TOMATO SAUCE**

(MUSSELS—APPROX. 24 TO 4 OZ.)
Mussels
2 crushed garlic cloves
1 T. olive oil
Crushed tomatoes (1 c. per 24 mussels)
Garlic powder
Oregano

COOK AS ABOVE STEAMERS. Lay shells on baking pan, cover with tomatoes and seasoning, bake 20 minutes in oven at 350°. Serve hot.

CHICKEN GALORE

- **CHICKEN AND HERBS**

($1/2$ CHICKEN = 1 PROTEIN)
2 pieces chicken (½ chicken)
Chopped fresh garlic
½ t. oregano
¼ t. thyme
½ t. sage
Parsley flakes
Onion flakes
1 T. olive oil
1 T. lemon juice
Dash paprika

TO PREPARE: Place chicken (skin side down) on a flat baking pan. Add 1/2 of the chopped garlic, sprinkle on the oregano, thyme, sage. Salt and pepper to taste. After 20 minutes in oven at 375°, turn chicken and lower heat to 325°. Add 1/2 cup of water and continue to bake for another 30 minutes. While chicken is cooking, mix the remainder of garlic and the parsley flakes, onion flakes, oil and lemon juice in cup. When chicken is ready, add the natural juice from pan into cup with herb sauce and pour over chicken. Sprinkle with paprika. Serve.

- **CHICKEN STEW**

(1 PROTEIN + 1 VEG.)
2 pieces chicken (1/2 chicken = 1 protein)
1/4 c. onion flakes
1/4 c. chopped green pepper
1/4 c. sliced mushrooms
1/4 c. diced carrots
1/8 t. fresh dill
1/2 t. sage
1/2 t. thyme
1/2 t. oregano
Salt and pepper

TO PREPARE: Just place everything in roaster on top of stove with cover. Cook on very low flame for 45 minutes. Serve hot. Delicious.

Proverb:
Solomon says: "Being cheerful keeps you healthy. It is slow death to be gloomy all the time."
*Am I cheerful or gloomy most of the time?

• ORIENTAL CHICKEN

(1 PROTEIN + 1 VEG.)
1 T. oil
½ c. sliced onion
¼ c. diced green pepper
¼ c. chopped celery
¼ c. bean sprouts
1 t. soy sauce
Garlic powder
Paprika
1½ chicken breasts, boned and cut into bite-size pieces
Salt and pepper
½ egg (beaten)

TO PREPARE: Use separate pans for chicken and vegetables. Use ½ oil to sauté vegetables, soy sauce, and spices. In separate pan, heat remainder of oil, add chicken, salt and pepper, egg, and stir on high flame. Turn and lower heat, and cook until tender. Pour chicken over vegetables. Raw vegetables cook down to about ½ the amount. Serve hot.

- **STUFFED WHOLE CHICKEN**

2 PORTIONS
(1 PROTEIN + 1 VEG.)
1 whole chicken (3 lbs.)
2 T. wheat germ
½ c. chopped celery
½ c. chopped mushrooms
½ packet onion soup
Rosemary
Sage
Thyme
Salt and pepper

TO PREPARE: Wash and salt chicken, mix vegetables with wheat germ and 2 T. cold water. Season and stuff chicken. Bake in oven for 1 hour at 325°. Cut in half and measure ½ of stuffing.

Today is the first day of the rest of your life.

• CHICKEN CACCIATORE

(FOR 4 PEOPLE OR 4 MEALS)
2 chickens (quartered or 8 pieces)
1 can crushed tomatoes (2 cups)
Basil
1 bay leaf
1 c. mushrooms
1 c. diced green pepper
1 c. diced celery
1 packet sweetener
¼ c. onion flakes
2 cloves crushed garlic
1 T. olive oil
Salt and pepper
Thyme
Garlic powder
Sage
Oregano

TO PREPARE: Place chicken in large pan skin side down. Bake in oven at 375°. After 15 minutes add ½ c. water. While chicken is cooking, prepare vegetables in pan on stove with medium flame. Mix tomatoes, basil, bay leaf, vegetables, sweetener, onion flakes, crushed garlic with oil, and sauté till tender. After chicken cooks 30 minutes in oven, turn and season with salt, pepper, thyme, garlic powder, sage, and oregano. Bake 15 minutes. Then pour vegetables over chicken and place in oven at 325° for 30 minutes. Take 2 pieces of chicken and measure 1 cup of vegetable and sauce mixture. Serve hot.

> *"Sometimes it takes a painful experience
> to make us change our ways."*
> KING SOLOMON

• CHICKEN AND BACON

(1 PROTEIN)
1 piece of chicken
2 slices bacon
2 T. onion flakes
Salt and pepper

TO PREPARE: Cook chicken on one side for 30 minutes, turn and bake for 10 minutes, sprinkle with onion flakes and seasoning, wrap in bacon, and finish cooking. Total time in oven at 350°, about one hour.

*I know that God wasn't punishing me,
He was conditioning me . . .*

*"Plan carefully and you will have plenty;
act too quickly and you will never have enough."*
                                    KING SOLOMON

HAMBURGER HAVEN

• HAMBURGER PATTY

(1 PROTEIN)
5 oz. raw chopped beef
1 t. onion soup mix
1 T. onion flakes
2 T. water
1 t. parsley flakes
1 t. Worcestershire sauce
Salt and pepper

TO PREPARE: Mix ingredients together, roll into ball, and flatten. Place in broiler for 10 minutes, turn, finish cooking. Yield: 1 4-oz. burger.

- **CHEESEBURGER**

(1 PROTEIN)

Same ingredients as above, just reduce amount of beef by one ounce to allow for ½ oz. of cheese added to top of burger 1 minute before done. Great with mustard and relish.

- **CHILI**

(1 PROTEIN + 1 VEG.)
4 oz. raw beef (ground)
1 T. oil
¼ c. onion flakes
1 t. chili powder
1 T. mustard
1 c. water
Garlic powder
1 c. crushed tomato
1 T. tomato paste
1 packet sweetener
Salt and pepper
¼ t. horseradish

TO PREPARE: Sauté beef in oil. Add other ingredients, stir, and cover. Reduce heat and cook for 35 minutes.

One compulsive bite is too much, then . . . a thousand aren't enough. All you have to worry about is the first. After that??

MEALS WITH VEAL

• VEAL AND PEPPERS (for 2)

(1 PROTEIN + ½ C. VEG.)
½ lb. veal cutlet cut in ½ inch strips
1 c. green diced peppers
1 T. oil
1 garlic clove, crushed
3 t. lemon juice
Dash rosemary
¼ c. onion flakes
Salt and pepper
½ packet sweetener
Dash thyme

TO PREPARE: Heat oil in large frying pan. Brown veal strips, then add other ingredients, stirring frequently for a couple of minutes on high flame. Reduce heat and cover. Cook until done, about 30 minutes. Delicious with ½ c. mushrooms.

"No man is an island." Find something bigger than yourself in which to believe.

• STUFFED VEAL ROLL

(1 PROTEIN + 1 VEG.)
1/4 c. sliced mushrooms
1/4 c. diced celery
1/4 c. onion flakes
2 T. tomato paste
Garlic powder
1 T. olive oil
Basil
1/4 c. diced tomatoes
1 T. wheat germ
2 T. parsley flakes
1/2 c. water
Salt and pepper
Thyme
Oregano
1 T. olive oil
2 slices of veal cutlet, 2 oz. each

TO PREPARE: Mix all ingredients (except veal and oil). Spoon onto slices of veal, roll, and tie. Place in hot oil in frying pan. Brown on high flame for several minutes, turning. Reduce heat, cover, cook another 30 minutes. Serve hot. Two rolls = 1 portion. You can refrigerate these rolls for a few hours and slice into wheels for a party.

The future is not so much determined by planning tomorrow as by acting today.

ROASTS

- **LEG O' LAMB**

(4 OZ. = 1 PROTEIN)
1 leg of lamb
1½ c. white vinegar
Juice of 2 lemons
Garlic cloves, sliced
Parsley flakes
Thyme
Salt and pepper
½ stick margarine
1 packet sweetener
Mint

TO PREPARE: The night before, marinate leg of lamb in 1½ c. vinegar and lemon juice. Cut slits in leg and fill with garlic. Rub on, by hand, all seasoning. Before cooking, rub on margarine. Place in roasting pan with 1 inch water in oven at 375°. Roast for a couple of hours. Keep basting. While lamb is in oven, prepare one cup of vinegar with sweetener and mint. Let stand. Weigh out 4 oz. lamb and spoon on desired amount of vinegar sauce. Serve hot or cold. Delicious.

Action is the Magic Wand.
Faith alone avails us nothing . . . Knowledge alone avails us nothing. You must act on the knowledge you have acquired. Remember, faith, thought, and action go hand in hand. Action is the magic wand and the time is now.

- **ROAST LONDON BROIL AND OYSTERS**

(4 OZ. = 1 PROTEIN)
London broil
12 plump oysters
Parsley flakes
Onion flakes
Salt and pepper
Thyme

TO PREPARE: Place meat in roaster; cut slits at top. Pour oysters on top; add seasoning. Cook until done, about 1 hour in oven at 375°. Cut very thin slices of meat to weigh 3 oz. and have a couple of oysters—1 oz. This is an interesting and wonderful combination.

Did you know that now *spelled backward is* won? *If I act positively now, what will I have won? Well, there's only my life, self-esteem, freedom, etc., etc., etc.*

---

4 Entertaining

Let's plan a party and have an international smorgasbord for our friends. You may choose . . .

First, what is more American than roast turkey, baked Virginia ham, and roast beef? Easy, too.
Next we'll have our Gefilte Fish (p. 30) and the Sweet and Sour Cold Fish (p. 29) on our table.
How about Leg o' Lamb (p. 46) and Stuffed Grape Leaves (p. 61).
We can offer Chicken Cacciatore (p. 40), our spaghetti (p. 62), and Mussels with Tomato Sauce (p. 36).
Don't forget Oriental Chicken (p. 38).
Round out the choice with Chili (p. 43).
Spinach and Mushroom Salad (p. 54).

Special Message
Again, I remind you that attitude is very important. Some compulsive overeaters may feel very uncomfortable with this kind of entertaining. I don't. Many of my friends can handle this without difficulty. If you feel uncomfortable with this, then by all means, avoid it. But before you criticize, remember, don't take my inventory. Food is a reality of life. "I can run, but I can't hide." I'm learning to cope with the realities of life one day at a time. And a reality is that there are times I am invited to parties or give them. I am part of this world and very happy to participate in social functions. The only thing I fear is "fear itself." I weigh and measure regardless of the situation, and God takes care of the rest.

"Not everything that you face can be changed, but nothing can be changed until you face it."

MENU I

APPETIZER: Seafood — 12 Mussels with Tomato Sauce (p. 36) = ½ protein & ¼ c. veg.

SALAD: Spinach and Mushroom — 2 cups with your choice of dressing (2 T. only) (p. 54)

MAIN COURSE: Chicken Cacciatore — 1 chicken breast plus ¾ c. of vegetable (p. 40)

DESSERT: Cup of Black 'n' Orange (p. 12) and conversation with happy, beautiful people

MENU II

APPETIZER: Stuffed celery with chicken liver: Weigh 1 oz. Chicken Liver Sauté (p. 26) and fill the ends of 2 celery stalks.

SALAD: Tossed green salad with dressing (2 T.) Measure out 1¾ cups. Allow ¼ cup for the celery used in the appetizer.

MAIN COURSE: Chicken and Herbs — 1 piece (p. 36)
VEGETABLE: String Beans Italian — ½ c. (p. 63)
Mushroom Magic — ½ c. (p. 59)

DESSERT: Cinnamon Coffee and conversation (p. 11)

Remember . . .
"This is your life, not a dress rehearsal."

*"If I can't have the things I want,
help me to want the things I can have."*

MENU III

APPETIZER:	Steamers 4 = 1 oz. protein (p. 35)
SALAD:	Cole Slaw — 2 cups (p. 56)
MAIN COURSE:	6 Mussels with Tomato Sauce = 1 oz. protein + 1/4 c. veg. (p. 36)
	Fish 'n' chips — 2 oz. = 1/2 protein and 1/4 c. veg. (p. 23)
VEGETABLE:	Brussels Sprouts 1/2 cup (p. 65)
DESSERT:	Espresso 'n' conversation

Abstinence is a privilege, so enjoy it!

MENU IV. CHEF'S SALAD

APPETIZER:	Pickled Mushrooms ½ c. (p. 59)
SALAD:	Mixed salad 2 c. + 2 T. Dressing
MAIN COURSE:	Rolled roast beef, turkey, ham, and cheese wheels (p. 81)
VEGETABLE:	Shoestring beets — ¼ c.
DESSERT:	Black coffee 'n' guess? No, try a little love.

"Fear is having faith in the wrong things."
What do you have faith in?

5
Salads and Vegetables

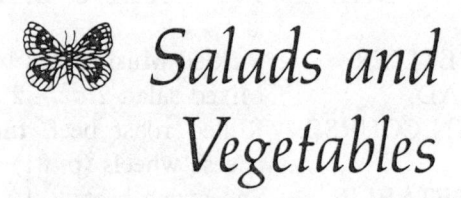

- **SPINACH AND MUSHROOM SALAD**
  (supper salad)

1 lb. chopped raw spinach
1 lb. snow-white cap mushrooms
1 small red onion
1 diced carrot
1/2 pack sweetener
Salt and pepper

TO PREPARE: Wash spinach and mushrooms thoroughly and drain. Spinach should be chopped into small pieces, and mushrooms sliced paper thin. Arrange in salad bowl, adding onion, sliced thin, and diced carrots. Sprinkle 1/2 packet sweetener, salt and pepper to taste. Measure out 2 full cups and 2 T. of your favorite dressing.

Try this dish as a main course by cooking bacon very crisp and weighing out 3 oz. Crumble and sprinkle over salad and add 1/2 oz. of your favorite grated hard cheese. This dish is your whole protein and supper salad equivalent.

• RAW GARDEN VEGETABLE SALAD

Cauliflower	Celery
Green beans	Scallions
Chickory	Carrots
Escarole	Shredded cabbage (red)
Mushrooms	Endive
Radishes	Cucumber

TO PREPARE: Chop, grate, shred all vegetables into very small pieces. Mix together, add salt, pepper to taste. Use 2 T. of your dressing on 2 cups of this salad. Different and delicious.

Put some of the undressed salad into a jar with 1/2 c. white vinegar, 1 packet sweetener, 1 t. mustard, 1 cinnamon stick, 1 clove. Cover and leave for 24 hrs. Very good for luncheons. Just remember to stop at one cup.

Today is the tomorrow you worried about yesterday.

---

56   SALADS AND VEGETABLES

- **COLE SLAW**

1 head cabbage
1/2 c. diced carrots
1/2 c. diced green pepper
1 c. diced celery
1/2 c. diced onion
1/2 c. pimento
2 packets sweetener
1 c. white vinegar
1 T. mustard
Salt and pepper

TO PREPARE: Soak cabbage and dry before using. Mix all vegetable ingredients in large bowl. Cabbage should be shredded very thin before adding to other ingredients. Next, pour vinegar, mustard and sweetener, into small bowl and mix. Use blender if available. Then pour over cole slaw, add salt and pepper to taste. Measure out 1 cup for lunch or 2 cups for supper salad. For supper, you may use 2 T. oil or other dressing to your liking.

- **CUCUMBER SALAD**

Cucumbers (not too large as they are seedy)
1 c. white vinegar
2 packets sweetener
Salt and pepper
Garlic powder

TO PREPARE: Slice cucumbers paper thin; soak overnight in salted water. Refrigerate. Drain just before using. Add vinegar, sweetener, and season to taste. One cup for lunch.

- **TOSSED GREEN SALAD**

1 head iceberg lettuce
½ head romaine
¼ head escarole
1 c. chopped celery
½ c. sliced onion
1 cucumber
1 c. cherry tomatoes
1 diced green pepper

TO PREPARE: Wash and dry all lettuce. Break into bite-sized pieces. Add other ingredients. Serve chilled with 2 T. dressing of your choice. Two cups for a delicious supper salad.

Think—A moment on the lips, forever on the hips.

Did you know that mushrooms and asparagus are nature's diuretic? All this and heaven too.

SALADS AND VEGETABLES

• ASPARAGUS VINAIGRETTE

(1 cup = 1 veg.)
1 lb. asparagus
2 t. lemon juice
1/4 c. parsley flakes
1/4 c. onion flakes
Salt and pepper
Dash of dill
1 c. wine vinegar

TO PREPARE: Cook asparagus till tender. Drain and refrigerate. After cooling add seasonings and vinegar. Refrigerate and serve chilled.

• FRESH COOKED ASPARAGUS

(1 cup = 1 veg.)
1 lb. asparagus
1 c. water
2 t. lemon juice
2 T. butter
Salt and pepper

TO PREPARE: Trim hard ends off asparagus. Lay flat in 1 c. of salted boiling water. Add lemon juice to bring out the flavor. Cook about 15 minutes. Serve hot. Pour melted butter over top. Add salt and pepper. Measure 1 c.

SALADS AND VEGETABLES

- **SKILLET MUSHROOM MAGIC**

(1 CUP = 1 VEG.)
1 lb. mushrooms
1 T. oil
1 clove garlic, crushed
1/4 c. diced green pepper
1/4 c. parsley flakes
Oregano
1/2 c. onion flakes
Salt and pepper

TO PREPARE: Trim ends off mushrooms. Wash and soak in salt water for 1/2 hour. Heat oil and crushed garlic in skillet. Add all remaining ingredients. Season. Cook 20 minutes. Serve hot.

"Share pain and it is lessened; share joy and it is multiplied."

- **PICKLED MUSHROOMS**

(1 CUP = 1 VEG.)
2 lbs. mushrooms
1/4 c. minced onion

SALADS AND VEGETABLES

1 bay leaf
1 cinnamon stick
½ c. pimento
2 c. white vinegar
1 T. mustard
1 clove
4 cloves garlic
Salt and pepper

TO PREPARE: Trim mushroom ends and boil for 10 minutes. Drain and chill. Leave whole or slice and place in large jar. Mix other ingredients in blender and pour over mushrooms. Cover tightly and let marinate in refrigerator at least overnight. Serve chilled.

- **MUSHROOMS AND TOMATO SAUCE**

(1 CUP = 1 VEG.)
1 lb. mushrooms
2 T. oil
2 t. lemon juice
1 can crushed tomatoes
Fresh dill
Oregano
½ packet sweetener
½ c. onion flakes
Garlic powder
Salt, pepper
Paprika

TO PREPARE: Trim mushroom ends. Wash and soak in salted water for ½ hour. Heat oil in skillet. Add mushrooms. Add lemon juice to bring out flavor of vegetables.

Pour in tomatoes, add seasonings, and simmer for 20 minutes. Serve hot.

Happiness is . . .
Looking down and seeing my feet . . .
Crossing my legs . . .
Getting closer to the people I like . . .
Not wearing tents . . .
Shopping, not settling . . .
Being asked . . .
Saying no when I want . . .
Looking in the mirror from the neck down . . .
Not having to buy in the fat person's shop . . .

- **STUFFED GRAPE LEAVES**

(1 CUP = 1 VEG.)
1 jar of marinated grape leaves
1/2 c. olive oil
1 c. onion flakes
1/2 c. diced green pepper
1/2 c. pimento
2 T. capers

62 SALADS AND VEGETABLES

½ c. chopped celery
1 packet sweetener
¼ t. oregano
½ t. rosemary
1 t. mint
1 t. fresh dill
1 t. salt
½ t. pepper
½ c. lemon juice

TO PREPARE: Wash grape leaves very carefully to remove any brine. Remove thick stem portions and cut large leaves in half. Soak in water for ½ hour. While leaves are soaking, heat olive oil in pan and on a low flame sauté all ingredients except herbs, spices, and lemon juice. Add herbs and spices and lemon juice. Cook for 10 minutes. Separate grape leaves and put one tablespoon of cooked filling in each leaf. Starting at base, fold over, fold in sides, rolling tightly toward point. Place in layers in pan with oil. Add 1 cup water and steam for 20 minutes. Put in refrigerator and serve cold. Measure out 1 cup, about 6 to a cup.

- **SPAGHETTI AND SAUCE**

(1 CUP = 1 VEG.)
1 T. oil
2 cloves garlic
1 16 oz. can crushed tomatoes
1 packet sweetener
⅛ c. basil
1 bay leaf
½ t. oregano

SALADS AND VEGETABLES

Salt and pepper
16 oz. can of French-cut string beans

TO PREPARE: In saucepan, heat oil and crushed garlic cloves. Add can of tomatoes and seasonings. Cook 30 minutes. Heat beans and measure 3/4 c. Pour 1/4 c. tomato sauce over them. Delicious.

I'm free. I have a choice of freedom and a freedom of choice. When I let go and let God, I'm free.

- **STRING BEANS ITALIAN**

(1 CUP = 1 VEG.)
1 lb. green beans
1 T. salt
2 T. olive oil
1 t. oregano
Salt and pepper
1 t. onion flakes
2 cloves garlic
1 t. red vinegar

TO PREPARE: Snip off tips of beans. Wash and soak in salt water about 1/2 hour. Boil 1 pt. water in large pot with 1 T. salt. Place beans in boiling water and cook till tender. Re-

SALADS AND VEGETABLES

move from heat and drain. Place in dish and add oil first and then seasonings. Chop garlic very fine, mix with the vinegar, and add. Serve hot or cold.

Life is a journey, not a destination. So, I will live each day as best I can. Please, join me. Together we won't get lost.

- **EXOTIC GREEN BEANS AND TOMATO SAUCE**

1 lb. cooked string beans (boil as above)
2 T. oil
1 c. onion flakes
1 small can crushed tomatoes
1 c. water
Salt and pepper
1 packet sweetener
1 t. basil
1 bay leaf, 1 sprig oregano, 1 clove, 1 cinnamon stick, 3 cloves of garlic all wrapped in a cloth sack and tied together

TO PREPARE: Heat oil in skillet and sauté onion flakes. Add can of tomatoes and 1 c. water. Add salt and pepper, sweetener, and basil. After sauce begins to bubble, lower heat and add sack of herbs and spices. Reduce heat and simmer with cover on low flame for 1/2 hour. Add string beans, which have been boiled till just a little tender. Finish cooking another 10 minutes without cover, stirring occasionally. The cinnamon stick gives off a very interesting flavor. Try it, you'll like it.

- **BRUSSELS SPROUTS**

(1 CUP = 1 VEG.)
1 lb. Brussels sprouts
1 T. salt
1 T. margarine
1/2 c. onion flakes
Salt and pepper
1 T. caraway seed (optional)
1 t. mustard (optional)

TO PREPARE: Soak sprouts in salt water for 15 minutes, cut off hard stems, and slit lengthwise. Place in boiling water with 1 T. salt, cover, and cook for 20 minutes. Remove from heat, drain, and add margarine and seasoning. Delicious hot or cold. When serving cold add a little vinegar.

Brussels sprouts may be used as a main course if you use your favorite cheese (2 oz.) shredded over top and placed in oven till cheese melts.

SALADS AND VEGETABLES

Look at me, I'm giving myself responsible love.

• CABBAGE PLAIN 'N' SIMPLE

(1 CUP = 1 VEG.)
1 head cabbage
Sweetener
Water
Salt and pepper to taste
2 t. lemon juice in boiling water

TO PREPARE: Soak cabbage in salt water for ½ hour. Quarter and place in 1 qt. boiling water. Cover and cook till tender, about 20 minutes. Remove from heat and drain. Add seasonings to taste. Lemon juice brings out flavor of vegetable while cooking.

• SWEET 'N' SOUR CABBAGE

(1 CUP = 1 VEG.)
1 head cabbage
¼ c. parsley flakes
Sweetener

Water
2 t. lemon juice in boiling water
1 c. white vinegar
1 t. caraway seeds (optional)

Soak cabbage in salt water for 30 minutes. Shred as for cole slaw. Place in boiling water with lemon to bring out flavor. Cook for 20 minutes, and drain. Mix parsley flakes, sweetener, and vinegar in cup and pour over cabbage. Add caraway seeds.

- **SAUERKRAUT, SO EASY**

(1 CUP = 1 VEG.)
1 16-oz. can sauerkraut
1 c. onion flakes
1 packet sweetener

TO PREPARE: Pour can of sauerkraut into saucepan with onion flakes and sugar substitute. Cover, and cook on very low flame for 20 minutes. The end result will be a pleasant surprise.

- **HUNGARIAN SAUERKRAUT**

(1 CUP = 1 VEG.)
1 16-oz. can sauerkraut
2 packets sweetener
1 packet onion-soup mix
2 c. water

SALADS AND VEGETABLES

½ can tomato paste
½ t. basil
Paprika
¼ c. onion flakes

TO PREPARE: Drain can of sauerkraut, place in skillet with other ingredients, and bake for 45 minutes in oven at 375°. Sprinkle paprika over top to give color. Serve hot with pork. Delicious.

"Hey, H.L., help me to get out of my own way so I'll be o.k."

• BROCCOLI WITH LEMON SAUCE

(1 CUP = 1 VEG.)
1 head broccoli
2 cloves garlic
3 t. lemon juice
Salt
1 T. melted margarine

TO PREPARE: Cut off hard ends and remove outer leaves. Soak for 30 minutes in salted water. Place in pot with 1 pt. boiling water (salted), stalks down. Remove and drain. Chop garlic very fine and mix through. Measure out 1 c.

and add lemon and margarine. Makes a main course when 2 oz. of cheese is shredded over top and melted in oven. Cheddar is especially good with broccoli.

- **CAULIFLOWER**

(1 CUP = 1 VEG.)
1 head cauliflower
1 T. melted margarine
Garlic powder
Salt and pepper
Parsley flakes
Paprika

TO PREPARE: Separate stems of cauliflower and soak in salted water for ½ hour. Place in boiling salted water and cook till tender, about 15 minutes. Remove, and add melted margarine, garlic powder, salt, pepper and parsley flakes, with paprika last.

This too, can be served as a main course with 2 oz. cheese melted over it. Try Swiss cheese with this. Very tasty.

- **CAULIFLOWER LASAGNE**

(1 VEG. + 1 PROTEIN)
Cauliflower (prepared as above)
3 oz. ricotta cheese
¼ c. tomato sauce
½ oz. grated cheese

TO PREPARE: Measure out ¾ cup chopped cauliflower, ¼ c. tomato sauce, 3 oz. ricotta, add ½ oz. of grated hard cheese. Put in blender and mix to fine consistency. Pour into small cup and bake for 20 minutes in oven at 350°. Delicious. Warning, make plenty for the family. It's *soooo* good.

Happiness is having the freedom of choice.
Are you giving yourself a choice?

• BAKED CAULIFLOWER AND CARROT

(½ OF 1 CUP VEG. + ½ OF ½ CUP VEG.)
½ c. boiled cauliflower, chopped
¼ c. diced cooked carrots
1 t. onion flakes
Salt and pepper
1 pat margarine, melted
Paprika

TO PREPARE: Measure ½ c. cooked chopped cauliflower and ¼ c. diced carrots. Put in blender with onion flakes, margarine, salt and pepper. Mix. Spoon into baking cup, bake for 10 minutes in oven at 350°. Add paprika last.

• CINNAMON CARROTS

(½ cup = 1 veg.)
1 bunch carrots
1 T. melted margarine
Salt and pepper
Parsley flakes
Cinnamon

TO PREPARE: Peel and wash carrots, and soak in salted water for 30 minutes. Cut in half lengthwise. Place in flat skillet in ½ cup water. Cover, and cook on very low flame until tender. Drain and add melted margarine, season, and garnish with parsley flakes. Sprinkle with cinnamon.

Abstinence makes the heart grow fonder!

• ZUCCHINI MEXICANA

(1 cup = 1 veg.)
1 T. olive oil
2 crushed garlic cloves
1 c. onion flakes
4 small zucchini
2 packets sweetener

Salt and pepper to taste
1 green pepper
Oregano
½ c. pimento
1 can crushed tomatoes
1 c. water
1 t. basil
1 dash Tabasco
1 t. horseradish
½ t. hot pepper
A few capers

TO PREPARE: Heat oil in large skillet. Brown garlic, add onion flakes and a little water. Cut zucchini into thin slices and place in skillet with one packet of sweetener and salt and pepper. Cook 5 minutes. Add diced green pepper, oregano, and pimento. Cook 5 minutes. Add tomatoes and 1 c. water, basil and other packet of sweetener. Lower heat, cover, simmer for 10 minutes, add the rest of the spices, and simmer for another 5 minutes. Careful when you eat it, it might bite back. It's hot and good.

Try this with 4 oz. of browned beef.

Follow recipe as above, mix in blender, pour into lettuce leaves, top with 2 oz. ground cooked beef and 1 oz. shredded cheese for Tacos.

• PEPPERS

(1 CUP = 1 VEG.)
4 red bell peppers (sweet)
1 T. olive oil
1 T. tomato paste

Salt and pepper
1 packet sweetener
Oregano

TO PREPARE: Cut peppers in half; remove seeds and stem. Soak in cold salted water for 15 minutes. Heat oil in skillet and put tomato paste and a little water on for about 2 minutes before laying the peppers flat in pan. Turn after 2 minutes, add seasoning, and lower heat. Cook until tender. Serve hot.

Peppers prepared as above may be served cold with a tablespoon of red vinegar added.

"I will not worry about tomorrow's rain and miss today's sunshine."

- **STEWED EGGPLANT**

(1 CUP = 1 VEG.)
1 large eggplant
1 c. crushed tomatoes
1 c. onion flakes
1 T. basil
Salt and pepper
1 packet sweetener
1 t. oregano
Garlic powder

74　SALADS AND VEGETABLES

TO PREPARE: Cut eggplant into bite-size pieces and place in refrigerator with a heavy dish pressing down overnight. This will remove the acid from this vegetable. Put all ingredients into saucepan and cover on low flame for 45 minutes. Serve.

Measure out one cup into small baking cup and add 2 oz. cheese and melt in oven for a main-course dish. Very tasty.

For variety try this with 3 oz. ricotta and ½ oz. grated hard cheese. Bake in oven for 10 minutes. Fast and easy lunch.

• WINTER SQUASH

(ONE SLICE = 1 VEG.)
1 acorn squash
Salt and pepper
Cinnamon (optional)
Sweetener (optional)
1 T. margarine

TO PREPARE: Wash the wax off green skin. Cut in half, remove seeds from center. Place on baking sheet skin side down. Bake in oven for 30 minutes at 350°. Remove and scoop out squash and put into blender with seasoning. Mash and serve as "sweet potato" by adding sweetener and cinnamon or just add margarine and put into baking dish in oven for 10 minutes.

- **STUFFED SQUASH**

(ONE SLICE = 1/2 CUP)
1 zucchini squash sliced into rings (1 inch wide)

TO PREPARE: Prepare as above only placing rings down on lightly greased baking sheet. Fill the center with 3 oz. meat filling (cooked chopped beef or sausage). Top that off with 1/2 oz. mozzarella just a minute before removing from oven. This is a delicious main course.

"I hope you have enjoyed some of these vegetable dishes as much as I have enjoyed sharing them with you."

6
Specialties: Desserts, "Free" Dressing, Relishes, Treats

- **BAKED APPLE FOR BREAKFAST**

(1 APPLE = 1 FRUIT)
Tart baking apples
2 t. lemon juice
Cinnamon
Black cherry diet soda or 1 packet sweetener (optional)

TO PREPARE: Prepare apples by washing. Leave skin on but remove core. Place in pan with 1 inch water. Top apples with cinnamon, lemon juice, diet soda or sweetener. Bake till juicy, about 45 minutes at 350°.

- **BAKED PINEAPPLE AND APPLE RINGS FOR BREAKFAST**

---

1 can pineapple slices packed in own juice
Tart baking apples
Sweetener, to taste

Ginger, to taste
Cinnamon, to taste

TO PREPARE: There are 5 slices to one cup of pineapple. Use 2½ slices. This will allow ½ apple. Dice the ½ slice pineapple and slice the ½ apple into 2 rings. Place the apple rings on top of pineapple slices. Put the ginger on the ½ diced slice pineapple and fill the centers of the whole slices of pineapple. Add cinnamon and sweetener. Place in one inch of water in open pan in oven at 375° for 30 minutes. You may use diet ginger ale in place of one inch of water.

- **MALTED**

(1 PORTION = ½ PROTEIN)
1 c. milk
4 ice cubes
Dash of vanilla flavoring
1 packet sweetener

TO PREPARE: Place in blender and whip until foamy.

- **STRAWBERRY MALT**

Same as above, add ½ c. strawberries. This is equivalent to ½ protein + ½ fruit.

• COFFEE-MAPLE WHIP

(ELIMINATE 1 OZ. PROTEIN)
1 envelope unflavored gelatin
4 oz. milk
2 c. hot black coffee
½ t. maple flavoring
2 packets sweetener
Dash of salt

TO PREPARE: Mix gelatin with cold milk to moisten. Dissolve in hot coffee. Add remainder of ingredients, and chill until it just begins to thicken. Then whip with hand mixer until it thickens. Mixture will increase considerably in volume. Spoon into dessert dish. Sprinkle on dash of cinnamon or nutmeg. For variety, try other flavorings.

• CUSTARD

(1 PROTEIN)
1 c. milk
Sweetener
1 egg
Nutmeg

TO PREPARE: Mix milk, sweetener, and egg. Pour into Pyrex baking cup. Sprinkle on nutmeg, bake at 350° for 50 minutes.

• EGGNOG

(1 PROTEIN)
1 c. milk
Dash nutmeg
1 egg
1 packet sweetener

TO PREPARE: Beat with rotary beater till foamy and serve.

• CHEESE CAKE

(4 OZ. = 1 PROTEIN)
3-lb. can ricotta cheese
2 envelopes unflavored gelatin
Dash salt
1 t. banana flavoring
1 egg
1 t. vanilla flavoring
1/4 c. lemon juice
Cinnamon, nutmeg, sweetener

TO PREPARE: Mix ingredients in blender, place in baking dish, and bake in oven at 375° for 45 minutes. Mixture should be soupy when you take it out. Chill a couple of hours in refrigerator and sprinkle on more sweetener.

SPECIALTIES

- **ONION DIP**

(½ PROTEIN)
½ c. plain yogurt
2 T. onion soup mix

TO PREPARE: Mix yogurt and soup mix and chill for at least one hour before serving. Very nice with raw vegetables eaten as finger salad.

- **DRESSING**

(FREE)
½ c. white vinegar
1 packet sweetener
Mint
1 T. mustard
Parsley flakes

TO PREPARE: Combine ingredients, shake well, and use with finger salad.

- **RELISH**

(2 VEGETABLES)
1 c. diced dill pickles
1 c. vinegar
Onion flakes
½ c. diced carrots
3 packets sweetener

TO PREPARE: Place pickles in blender. Add other ingredients. Put in jar with cinnamon stick and clove, and shut tight. Let marinate at least 24 hours. Eliminate appropriate amount of vegetable for amount used.

With Discipline . . . We Can!

- **DIET CATSUP**

(FREE)
1 can tomato sauce (unsweetened)
1 t. garlic powder
3 packets sweetener
¼ c. red vinegar
Salt

TO PREPARE: Bring ingredients to boil and simmer till thick. Chill.

- **PARTY WHEELS**

(1 PROTEIN)
1 slice roast beef or 1 oz.
1 slice turkey or 1 oz.
1 slice baked ham or 1 oz.
1 slice Swiss cheese or ½ oz.

SPECIALTIES

TO PREPARE: First lay out the slice of roast beef, then place the turkey, the ham, and the cheese on top, in that order. You now should have the ingredients in one even stack. Begin at the end closest to you and roll away from you into long roll. Roast beef should be outer layer. Holding firmly, cut into four even wheels and put toothpick through each wheel to hold it together. The end result will be very pretty. This is a nice way to serve cold cuts on a chef's salad.

Food was never my problem, just my misuse of it was. So here I am using food to sustain me, not abuse myself. I hope I have done a service for you by writing this book. If not, there was a need in me and I took action.

It must be right for me, 'cause I feel real good.
Love,
Lady Anne

7

Just for Today

Date _____

I WILL EAT:

BREAKFAST

    Fruit _____

    Protein _____

    Beverage _____

LUNCH

    Protein _____

    Finger Salad _____

    Vegetable _____

    Beverage _____

DINNER

    Protein _____

    Vegetable _____

    Beverage _____

Use as sample to write down your food commitment each day . . . everyday.

Abstinence from compulsive eating is the most important thing in your life!

8
The Butterfly Story

Whenever we see a fuzzy caterpillar, it is hard to believe that someday this ugly, crawling little creature will soar on wings as bright as any flower.

Before this change comes about, the fuzzy little worm withdraws from its caterpillar world, finds itself a place alone, and painfully, with much struggling, wraps itself tightly into a cocoon of its own making; it seals itself off from the world. Time passes, and gradually, a crevice appears in its hard outer layer, and finally a new creature emerges, quite a different little creature too. It begins to flutter its wings and become familiar with its new surroundings, going from flower to flower gathering up strength from each and at the same time leaving the pollen that it has gathered up from every other flower it has visited—thus enabling the flowers to make seeds and be born again.

THE BUTTERFLY STORY

Compulsive overeaters have much in common with the butterfly. Time was when we were unlovely creatures too. Then we find a program of recovery, others with the same disease. We share with each other and gather strength and hope. Soon we come out of our little "cage" into the light. We, too, go through our growing pains and emerge very different creatures.

Then we carry to others what we have found, and as we go to others, we are strengthened by them, and in turn, we leave with each one some of what all the others have given to us.

The butterfly is a spiritual symbol. It represents transformation, beauty, fragility, and has been described as the "Kiss of God."

The butterfly surrenders to change and emerges beautiful and free. The compulsive overeater surrenders to a program, is reborn, and a "butterfly" emerges . . . and Butterflies Are Free.

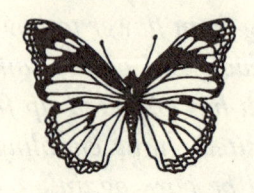